64 DIY natural beauty recipes

How to Make Amazing Homemade Skin Care Recipes, Essential Oils, Body Care Products and More

Jane Moore

Table of Contents

Natural Recipes for Moisturizing

Natural Recipes for Exfoliating

Hair Shampoo and Conditioner

You Are Ready to Make it Your Own

Bonus Recipes

74 - Hair Mousse for Healthy Curls

Taking Care of Your Skin Naturally

Feeling good is important, but so is looking your best. For many us the idea of using unnatural products and putting chemicals onto our skin is unappealing. Instead, you'd prefer to find a more natural way to take good care of your skin. After all, why can't we choose natural options?

Great news – you can! We are going to give you 64 natural skin care recipes that you can make yourself. All of them are easy to create and most of the ingredients you need to make these recipes, you'll find in your kitchen.

You can buy organic or natural skin care products, but why bother when you can make your own for a fraction of the cost, and then you know exactly what you are putting on your skin. You can tweak recipes so they are perfect for you. For example, perhaps you don't like rose, then switch rose for lavender, or perhaps you like a certain brand of shea butter then you can choose to use that brand.

You are about to discover 64 natural recipes that you can use to keep your skin looking beautiful regardless of your age. In the following pages, we will introduce you to a different way of taking care of your skin and to age beautifully – it's not a new way; it's actually an old way, following the timeless principles of generations before you. It seems that when it comes to skin care, there are some powerful lessons to be learned.

How did previously generations manage to age beautifully when it seems today, we struggle with that very concept? Earlier generations were wise and they were able to age beautifully, without all the fancy skin care products that we have at our disposal today. Today, aging is a billion dollar industry and honestly, many of the products that we buy, in an effort to look our very best, simply don't work and many actually pose a health risk. So instead, let's explore a more natural way.

Are you ready? Let's get started. By the end of this book, you'll have 64 DIY natural recipes that you can quickly and easily create.

A Word of Caution

For the most part creating your own beauty products couldn't be safer. However, you should be cautious of allergies. If you have not used a particular ingredient in the past, it is always a good idea to do a skin test to make sure you have no allergic reaction.

Also, if you are pregnant some essential oils can pose a health risk. Be familiar with what your physician considers safe during your pregnancy.

Aging Beautifully – Bases for Natural Skin Care

Women want to have beautiful glowing skin and men

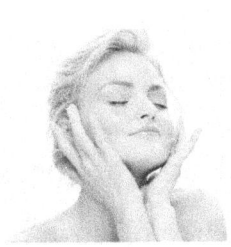

appreciate this beauty. In fact, the modern day man also works hard to keep his skin healthy and looking great. We are hardwired to be attracted to people with clear skin and a glowing complexion, because it represents good health. Today, more than ever, it's important to look back and see what we can learn from the way our ancestors cared for their skin in a more natural, healthier manner.

Honey Skin Care

Earlier generations used honey for many things besides cooking, which included skin care. We could certainly learn from some of these earlier practices. Honey is powerful antioxidant and anti-microbial, and it does an excellent job of absorbing and retaining moisture. Honey protects the skin from UVA and UVB rays and it also rejuvenates your skin. Many natural beauty cosmetics and skin care products contain honey.

Honey is a humectant. This means it draws and binds water from the air into your skin. A honey mask is an excellent skin treatment. To hydrate and soften your skin, apply it to slightly damp skin and leave it on for 15 to 30 minutes. You can use it daily if you like.

Honey is also an excellent cleanser. Take a single drop of honey and mix it with water in the palm of your hand. Then cleanse your face like you would with any cleanser. Finish by rinsing.

Honey has long been used to treat sunburn and today it still is an excellent choice to soothe your sunburn.

Honey is readily available to use and it is very affordable.

Shea Butter Skin Care

Shea butter comes from the shea nut tree, which grows in Africa. The shea nut tree contains a nut, which is crushed, dried and then ground. The resulting powder is then boiled, releasing a green substance that rises to the top. Once this solidifies, you have shea butter.

The use of shea butter for skin care is not new. For centuries, women in Africa have been using shea butter to moisturize their skin and protect it from the sun, wind and salt water. It has a natural SPF equivalent of 3.

Shea butter is unique because it has a high fat content, and it is very high in Vitamins E, A, and F. All of these work together to improve cell generation.

Shea butter is one of the natural ingredients commonly found in many different skin care products because of these superior qualities. High-end cosmetics use shea butter, because of its emollient properties, moisturizing properties and its ability to penetrate the skin.

Shea butter can also be used to treat dermatitis, eczema, burns, scars, rashes, dark spots, blemishes, skin discolorations, severely dry skin and to reduce wrinkles.

You can also use shea butter to moisturize your dry scalp and stimulate hair growth. It is commonly found in hair conditioners, as it is exceptionally good at adding moisture to dry brittle hair and preventing breakage.

The only problem with commercial products is that even though they may contain shea butter, it could still contain chemicals, so you need to carefully read labels to ensure you get the full benefits of shea butter in a natural, chemical free product. It has no toxicity, so it is an excellent choice for skin care.

Shea butter has a shelf life of 2 years and it needs to be stored in a cool place. Our ancestors have long known the true value of this unique nut. Now you can experience its skin benefits too.

Jojoba Skin Care

Jojoba comes from the Simmondsia Chinensis plant, which is a small shrub that grows in some areas of Mexico and Arizona. The benefits of jojoba oil have long been known and it reaches far beyond skin care. It can be used to treat burns, insect bites, stretch marks and a number of other skin issues.

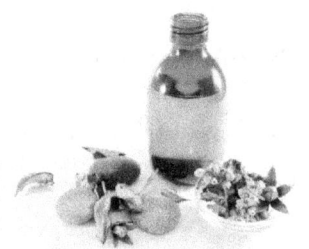

The cosmetic industry likes jojoba, and believes it to be one of the best ingredients in the world to use in cosmetics. It is also used in many natural moisturizers and anti aging skin care products. Jojoba is commonly referred to as the miracle oil.

While it is called jojoba oil, it is not actually an oil. It is a botanical extract. It was during the 1930's that chemists first discovered jojoba was actually 98 percent pure liquid wax ester, with properties that resemble the sebum the human body produces for the skin. The only other place this has ever been found is in sperm whale oil. The jojoba plant grows easily, so the oil is readily available.

Jojoba oil is quickly absorbed by the skin and does not leave an oily residue. If it is used daily as a moisturizer, it softens and protects the skin, keeping it youthful and supple. You can use it on your entire body. It is non clogging (non-comedogenic), so it is also an excellent treatment for acne. It is also an excellent makeup remover and lip balm.

Studies have shown if your skin is already showing signs of aging, when jojoba oil is continually used as a moisturizer, it can decrease the look of fine lines and wrinkles by as much as 26%.

Aloe Vera Skin Care

Aloe has been used to treat wounds and burns right back to our caveman days. There is a great deal of science behind aloe vera that shows the gel can help boost your immune system function and destroy cancer tumors.

Aloe also plays an important role in helping us age slower and more gracefully. Most people are only aware of the topical uses of aloe, but our ancestors were much wiser and relied on aloe for many different uses.

Aloe vera comes from the succulent aloe plant, which grows in the desert and during rainy periods swells to 130% of its normal

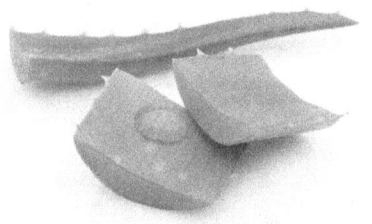

size as it draws in water. During the dry periods, they slowly start shrinking back to the size to begin with and all the water they consumed gets locked in the gel inside the aloe leaves. This is the potent gel we use. It is packed with all kinds of minerals, amino acids, vitamins, enzymes and antioxidants that fight off free radicals.

Aloe vera is close to the skin's PH so it will balance all skin types. It will also create elastin and collagen, which keeps your skin looking younger. Aloe vera opens up your skin's pores so they are better able to receive nutrients like moisturizer when you are dehydrated.

Keep it Simple

Far too many of the skin care and beauty products on the market contain carcinogens and chemicals that interrupt the endocrine system, which is associated with a number of cancers including breast cancer.

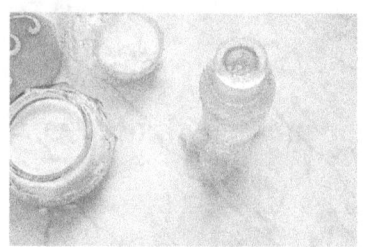

Why not keep it simple and choose products with natural ingredients. Ask yourself, which skin care and cosmetics you must use, and what are the healthiest alternatives you can find. Use the fewest products possible and then choose natural. We're going to share 64 natural skin care recipes you can do yourself, which will give you more control over what products you put on your skin.

Why You Should Choose Natural Skin Care

There are many benefits when you use natural skin care products. Natural skin care will provide you with the smoothest, softest, healthiest skin possible. When used regularly, it can postpone and even reverse the aging process.

Natural skin care is a healthier choice. There are not the risks associated with the use of chemical skin care products. If you are planning to use a commercial product, you should always read the ingredients before you decide to use it.

You also need to use a little caution because labels can be deceiving. The FDA does not regulate the chemical ingredients in skin care products. Aging beautiful doesn't have to be complicated.

The Benefits of Natural Beauty Products

The beauty industry is kind of like the wild-wild west. Because it is unregulated, there are toxic chemicals floating around in beauty products we use every day. This includes skin care products, cosmetics, personal hygiene products and other beauty products. These products can pose a real risk and sadly,

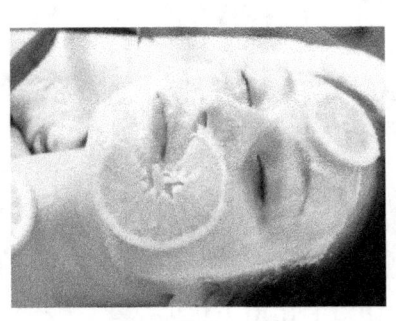

it may be years before we are aware that there is a health concern with any of these ingredients.

Instead of risking your health that chemicals could cause, look for natural beauty products or, better yet, make your own homemade beauty products using common kitchen ingredients. When you buy products, watch for the empty natural claims that are made far too often. Don't just believe what is on the packaging. The words 'organic' and 'natural' are two of the most misused words in the cosmetic and beauty industry.

In the US, a USDA certified organic seal means at least 95 percent of the ingredients are organic, but remember that other 5 percent of ingredients could contain harmful synthetics.

Read Labels for Words Your Recognize

Look for words you are familiar with lavender, aloe vera, ylang, vitamin E, vitamin A and the list goes on. Here's a rule, you can live by - if you can't pronounce the words listed on the ingredients then it is likely they are synthetic chemicals. Words such as DMDM or PEG should be a warning, as these ingredients don't belong on your skin if you want to age beautifully. You should also avoid synthetic fragrances, 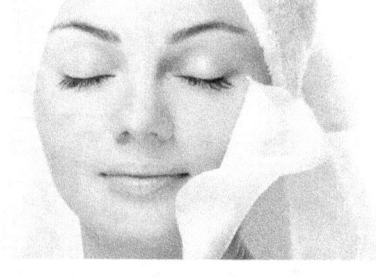 which are made up of hundreds of chemicals and toxic phthalates.

Have you ever noticed that the woman who use the most skin products and cosmetics, and who have the longest skin care regime, often also have the most wrinkles? That's because long-term use has the potential to age your skin faster. Women who use the least amount of products and/or natural products tend to age slowly. Of course, genetics plays a role, as do lifestyles. There's also, no study to back this, but just a general observation. You would think that the women who used these expensive, commercial formulas would be the ones that aged the slowest.

The reason that they tend to age faster is likely linked to two things - the chemicals in the products they use and the results they see aren't real. For example, product A is applied and wrinkles seem to disappear, but it's the result of a chemical reaction, not because the skin has actually been healed or became healthier. What's even more concerning is the number of these ingredients that are known as cancer causing carcinogens.

Avoid the Top Offenders

You should avoid many different ingredients because of the potential health risks and the direct link to cancer. Why not opt for healthier natural choices? Here are some things to avoid:

- Anti-aging creams containing lactic, BHA acids, AHA acids, glycolic, etc.
- Heavily scented products
- Liquid hand soaps that contain triclosan/triclocarban
- Moisturizers and creams containing petrolatum, PAHs, etc.
- Nail polish and nail polish removers with formaldehyde, DBP, toluene, etc.
- Shaving creams, hair spray, hair gels, and hair dyes that contain isobutene, nonylphenol, fungicides, etc.
- Skin lighteners containing hydroquinone
- Sunscreens containing chemicals that mimic estrogen

Disguised Chemicals

When you use skin care products containing chemicals, your skin cannot filter out the toxins and impurities. Natural skin care is much gentler on your skin and it also nourishes the skin.

The Oxford Dictionary defines natural as, *"existing in, or caused by nature; not artificial; uncultivated; wild existing in natural state; not disguised or altered."*

The definition is very clear, yet the beauty industry that has managed to stretch the meaning of the word 'natural' to something that you can't recognize.

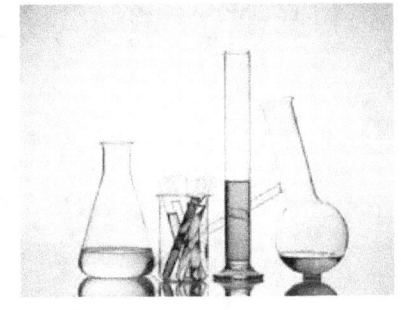

Pick up one of these products marked 'natural' and read the label – what you will often find is a long list of chemical names, and then the words "derived from (insert natural substance)." You would think this meant it was referring to a natural ingredient(s), but nothing could be further from the truth. It is very misleading.

Let's look at an example. The ingredient "Sodium Hydroxysultaine" is listed and then it reads, "Derived from coconut oil." This might make you think that somehow these chemicals are natural. Rarely is this true, and in the few instances when it is, chemical solvents are used to extract the natural ingredient. There is absolutely nothing natural about the process or the ingredients.

Organic Skin Care

Organic is different from natural. The Oxford dictionary defines organic as *"produced and involving production without the use of pesticides, artificial fertilizers or synthetic chemicals."*

Seems pretty straightforward right? Wrong! The trouble is the beauty industry plays on and manipulates the words taking the meaning completely out of context.

Let's look at an example. Have a look at your shampoo bottle. You'll likely see the ingredient Cocamide DEA on the list of ingredients. This is what foaming agent in your shampoo. To create this ingredient requires Diethanolamine - DEA to be added, which is a known 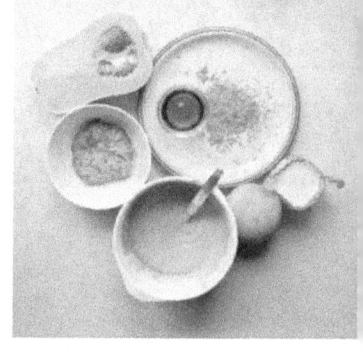 carcinogen. This means even if every other ingredient is natural or organic the product is not natural and it may pose a health risk.

If you see a label that reads organic, you assume it has no chemicals. That's exactly what deceitful companies want you to think. These companies use the chemistry based definition for organic, which reads *"a compound that contains a carbon atom."* For the consumer this creates confusion.

Let's look at an example. Let's say a company uses "Methyl Paraben," which is a petrochemical preservative that is highly toxic. They will call it organic. How can they do this? They can do this because it comes from rotting leaves that over thousands of years, have turned into crude oil, which is what the company uses to make the preservative. You see the word organic and think natural and pure and that's not always so.

The problem is that there are no regulations on how the term organic can be used unless it is 'certified organic,' which is regulated by numerous different agencies around the world. If you buy "certified organic," you can be sure of the authenticity of what's in the skin care product is actually organic.

Emollients

Emollients protect your skin by creating a barrier and preventing dryness. They are also a healing agent. Water is the best emollient there is. However, it evaporates quickly so its effectiveness is minimal. When emollient oils, called emulsions, are used to hold it to the skin, it can be very effective.

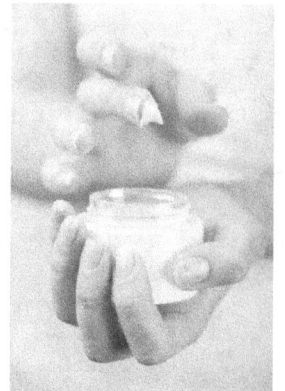

Synthetic emollients coat the skin just as if you were wrapping your skin in a plastic wrap. This means it can't breathe or perspire and this can irritate the skin. Some of these toxic synthetic emollients will accumulate in the lymph nodes and the liver with the potential for serious health concerns. They are also not biodegradable, so this has a negative effect on the environment.

Natural emollients are a better choice, because they nourish the skin. The skin's enzymes can metabolize natural emollients and absorb them. Natural emollients are both edible and biodegradable.

4 Natural Emollients

These are powerful natural emollients you should be aware of.

1. **Avocado** – This is a natural way to nurture your skin without chemicals. Avocado is rich in essential nutrients that soothe and moisturize your skin. Avocado will 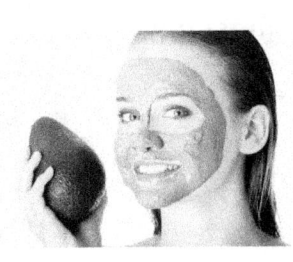 reduce fine lines and wrinkles to help you age beautifully.

2. **Shea Butter** – It is extracted from the shea nut kernels. This oil is actually edible and it is very soothing to your skin. It can really help to protect your skin during the harsh winter months.

3. **Rosehip** – It can help to reduce wrinkles, heal burns and eczema, and reduce scars. Rosehip oil has significant anti aging qualities and it will give your skin a youthful glow.

4. **Jojoba Butter** – An excellent skin moisturizer that is very similar to human sebum, so it protects the skin. It doesn't feel greasy or oily and is excellent is the slowing the aging process.

4 Synthetic Emollients You Should Avoid

Synthetic emollients are made from chemicals and are in many of the skin care products on the market. These are some of the most common synthetic emollients you should avoid.

1. **Synthetic alcohols** –If the ingredients include any of these phrases, you should avoid using: Butyl, Benzyl, Propylene, Cetearyl, Myristyl propyl, Cetyl, Glyceryl, or Isopropyl.
2. **PEG compounds** - May contain the toxic by-product dioxane (i.e. PEG- 45 Almond Glyceride)
3. **Hydrocarbons** - Contains carcinogenic and mutagenic Polycyclic Aromatic Hydrocarbons (PAHs).
4. **Silicone Oils** - This is the equivalent of wrapping your skin in plastic. It results in clogged pores and it is said to cause tumors when applied to the bodies of test animals. They include chemicals like cyclomethycaine, copolyol, or dimethicone.

Humectants

A cream is supposed to keep the skin moist. A great many creams do this by creating a suffocating film that stops the loss of moisture from your skin. Natural humectants like glycerin will pull water from the surrounding air into the skin's tissue to

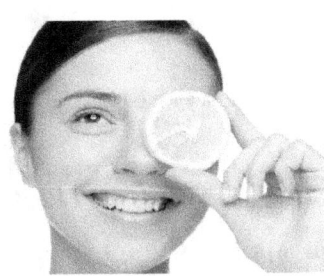

keep your skin moist. However, there needs to be moisture in the air or on your skin for humectants to be effective.

Elastin, keratin and collagen are three popular humectants that will put a protective film on the skin. Generally, they come from animals. Some manufacturers are proclaiming you can use certain animal proteins to revitalize aging cells – to even replace these cells. There is no science to back up this bold claim.

Even when these molecules are broken down, they are still too big to be able to enter the skin. If somehow they do penetrate your skin, your immune system would reject them as a foreign object.

Lecithin, which is an excellent humectants, provides natural phospholipids that attract water from the surrounding air and then hold that water in areas of your skin needing hydration.

Our environment, including things like the wind, sun and pollution, along with detergents and chemicals found in the majority of skin cleansers will strip away our natural phospholipids from the top skin layer leaving it looking rough to the naked eye.

Your top skin layer is a protective barrier and it no longer metabolizes the phospholipids that are in your top layer of the skin, so it is not replaced with your natural cell function. However, a recent study found that when plant phospholipids were topically applied the skin's barrier function was restored and protected from harmful substances.

3 Natural Humectants to Look For

Humectants are commonly found in skin care products. Avoid the chemicals and look for these three much safer choices. Ironically, they actually work better than chemicals do. In fact, our ancestors would have found these in their natural plant form.

1. **Lecithin** – Is a natural moisturizer derived from soybeans that can penetrate the epidermis and reach the cell level.

2. **Panthenol (pro-vitamin B5)** – It is a natural anti-inflammatory with anti itching qualities that is easily absorbed by the skin. It is very effective in treating acne.

3. **Glycerin** - Used as a moisturizer for dry and rough skin. Various studies found glycerin has strong humectant properties.

3 Synthetic Humectants to Avoid

Synthetic humectants are made from chemicals and these chemicals have a range of side effects ranging from mild to very serious, and some are even linked to cancer.

1. **PEG compounds** (i.e. Polyethylene Glycol) – May contain the highly toxic by-product dioxane.

2. **Propylene Glycol** – It is an irritant and it can cause contact dermatitis. It is also linked to some cancers.

3. **Ethylene/Diethylene Glycol** – It is an irritant and it can cause contact dermatitis.

Emulsifiers

Emulsifiers hold the ingredients together that would normally
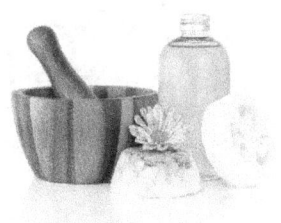 repel each other. Emulsifiers are often found in products that need to be shaken. Synthetic emulsifiers are usually petroleum based or hydrocarbon derivatives, and they are common allergens.

5 Natural Emulsifiers to Look For

Rather than choosing the popular chemical emulsifiers, here are 5 natural emulsifiers you can look for.

1. **Candelilla** – This wax is therapeutic in treating skin inflammation and it is an effective anti-inflammatory treatment for skin disorders.
2. **Jojoba** – It is an excellent skin moisturizer that is very similar to the human sebum, so it protects the skin really well without feeling greasy or oily. It offers a great deal of beauty value in the aging process.

3. **Quince Seed** - Is one of the oldest cultivated herbs, and it has excellent moisture retaining and skin renewing benefits.
4. **Rice Bran** – A natural antioxidants and it is hypoallergenic. It is a small molecule so it can easily penetrate the skin.

4 Synthetic Emulsifiers to Avoid

Synthetic emulsifiers are usually based on harmful chemicals. If you are unsure if something is chemical, chances are if you can't pronounce it, it is. Here are four of the most common synthetic emulsifiers to avoid

1. Alkoxylated Amides (can turn into carcinogens in the body).
2. Laurate, Isopropyl Stearate, Palmitate, Oleate, etc.
3. PEG Compounds (may contain the toxin dioxane).
4. Silicone, Ozokerite, Ceresin, and Montan Waxes.

Surfactants

Surfactants are agents that work on the surface of the skin to dissolve the oils that hold dirt, and you can use water to rinse them away. This is why they are found in the majority of skin cleansers and shampoos. However, these surfactants often contain the carcinogen dioxin.

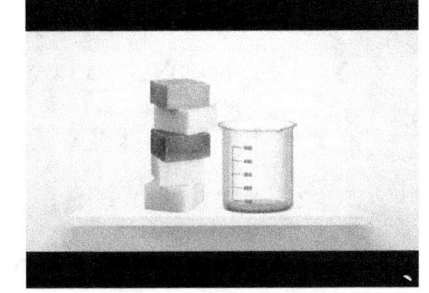

This same carcinogen was sprayed during Agent Orange in the Vietnam jungle. It was responsible thousands upon thousands of birth defects and cancers within the Vietnamese population and a significant increase in cancer rates in Australian and USA military personnel that sprayed the agent.

Natural foaming agents are a safer choice. They will cleanse your skin and hair without stripping away important natural oils, and you won't die from using them.

4 Natural Surfactants to Look For

A much better option to chemicals is to choose a natural surfactant. These natural surfactants won't cause cancer or age your skin. They will help you age beautifully while feeling fresh and clean.

1. **Yucca Extract** – It heals the skin and the high saponin gives it its soapy texture. In shampoo, it adds volume and shine.

2. **Soapwort** – It cures skin problems like acne, psoriasis, eczema, boils, etc. Rich in saponins makes it nature's cleansing agents.

3. **Quillaja Bark Extract** – It acts as a foaming agent and it is a terrific option over synthetic surfactant. There are many plants have natural surfactants.

4. **Castile Soap** – Made from 100% olive oil, Castile soap is gentle and great for your skin. The Squalene helps your skin to retain moisture.

6 Synthetic Surfactants to Avoid

These foaming agents make you feel like your skin care or shampoo is working great while your health is put at risk. There are many synthetic surfactants, but there are 6 of the most common synthetic surfactants.

1. DEA compounds.
2. Dioctyl Sulfosuccinate.

3. PEG (Polyethylene Glycol) compounds.

4. Ingredient containing Lauryl in the name.

5. Ingredient containing Sulphate in the name.

6. Ingredient containing Sodium in the name.

Preservatives

Just like your food deteriorates and spoils, it is natural for skin care and beauty products to deteriorate and decay over time. This happens when you use natural skin care containing natural preservatives.

On the other hand, synthetic preservatives made from chemicals, which are very effective at preserving products, have not been proven to be safe, so you may want to reconsider if you want to put these products on your skin. It's better to avoid synthetic preservative and look for natural ones that are proven to help you age beautifully.

4 Natural Preservatives to Look For

1. **Vitamin E** (D-Alpha Tocopherol Acetate) – It is an excellent preservative and healing agent with antioxidant properties.
2. **Tea Tree Essential Oil** – Is great for your skin, and it has anti-viral and anti-fungal benefits, which makes it a perfect preservative to use in skin care and hair care.
3. **Thyme Essential Oil** - An excellent preservative and it has anti fungal and anti viral properties.

4. **Grapefruit Seed Extract** –An excellent preservative and it has anti fungal and anti viral properties.

A number of people think synthetic chemicals are safe when applied to the skin. They are sold to us based on hype and false promises, but the truth is that they are linked to countless side effects, reactions, and in some cases death. Some have done a great deal of damage before they are pulled off the market.

Mother Nature knows best. You will be much better trying to live in harmony with nature, rather than trying to control it, because when we try to control it, we always pay dearly. Sadly, far too many of us will be diagnosed with a deadly form of cancer. In the US, 1 in 3 will be diagnosed with cancer. It is in the interest of your health that you avoid toxic synthetic chemicals every opportunity you can.

10 Synthetic Preservatives to Avoid

These synthetic preservatives are chemicals and often cause allergic reactions. Worse, they are very toxic.

1. Quarternium-15.
2. Propyl, Methyl, Butyl.
3. Methylisothiazolinone/Methylchloroisothiazolinone.

4. Isothiazolinone.

5. Imidiazolidinyl Urea (Germall 115) and Diazolidinyl Urea (Germall II).

6. Ethyl.

7. Butylated Hydroxytoluene.

8. Butylated Hydroxyanisole (BHA).

9. 3-diol, Bronopol.

10. 2-Bromo-2-Nitro-Propane-1.

This mix of synthetic chemicals is used in many skin care products and cosmetics. It is alarming, because these same chemicals have been linked directly to the huge increase in cancer rates in North America and other developed parts of the world. These are cancers our ancestors did not experience, who instead relied on nature for their preservatives. Some of these preservatives actually speed up the aging process. Ironic, since they are often found in anti aging products.

The Health Benefits of Beeswax

Beeswax is secreted from the worker bees wax glands, which are on the underside of her abdomen. When honey is harvested, the top layer of wax is scraped off to reveal the honey.

Beeswax's non-allergenic properties make it a good skin protector. The North Carolina State University found beeswax slows down the disbursement of medication in the body and nourishes your skin. It has antibacterial, germicidal, antioxidant and anti-allergenic qualities, which are all very powerful qualities.

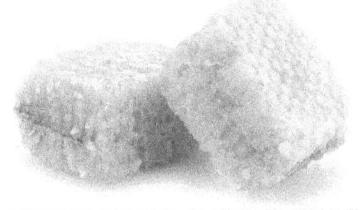 It is a great choice in natural skin care products and lip balms, because it contains natural moisturizers. Beeswax locks in moisture and keeps your skin firm. It helps the skin heal. According to the Bastyr Center for Natural Health, you can mix beeswax with other products, such as honey or olive oil, to produce lotions or balms, which are excellent eczema and psoriasis remedies.

The qualities of beeswax make it highly desirable in skin care products and in nourishing the skin to slow down the aging process.

The Use of Essential Oils

Our ancestors used essential oils. Today, essential oils continue to play an important role in natural skin care products and natural cosmetics. They offer a beautiful fragrance, offer a number of health qualities and play an integral role aiding with the aging process.

Let's have a look at some of the most common ones.

- **Ylang Ylang**

  On the skin, ylang-ylang oil is extremely soothing and its balancing action means it works well on all skin types. It stimulates effect on the scalp, resulting in luxurious hair growth. Pamper yourself with skin care products containing ylang ylang.

- **Orange**

  When orange is used in a lotion or cream it will help the lymphatic system, and to detoxify congested skin. It makes an excellent general skin tonic and it works well for more mature skin, dermatitis, acne and to soothe dry skin that is irritated. The tonic action stems from the action it has in supporting the skin's collagen formation, which is necessary for healthy, younger looking skin and aging beautifully.

- **Lemon Oil**

  Lemon oil benefits your circulatory system. It helps to clear acne, remove dead skin cells, clean greasy skin and hair and slow the aging process. Lemon oil can be used in a cream or lotion on the skin. The astringent properties are excellent for oily skin conditions.

- **Lavender**

  Lavender is a highly therapeutic essential oil used to treat oily skin, acne, dermatitis, burns and scars. It is a powerful analgesic, antiseptic and anti-inflammatory. Lavender helps you age beautifully, and you'll smell so nice too.

- **Jasmine**

  Jasmine oil tones dry, greasy, irritated and sensitive skin reduce scarring and stretch marks, increases skin elasticity. It is used in skin care products to improve elasticity and calm irritated skin.

  Jasmine is one of the most expensive oils because it is difficult to extract. It takes approx. 8 million handpicked jasmine blossoms to produce 1 kilogram of essential oil. Jasmine is picked at night when their aroma is most powerful.

Thankfully, it does not require a lot of jasmine in a product because it is highly concentrated, which makes it affordable, and certainly worth the cost.

Essential oils can help us age beautifully, but also in all their other uses, because aging beautifully is more than skin deep.

Essential oils are used to rejuvenate, restore and improve the appearance of aging and wrinkled skin. Numerous studies have shown that essential oils can improve skin conditions like acne, eczema, dry skin, freckles and clogged pores.

Essential Oil Cautions

In some cases, it is better to not use essential oils at all. Don't use any oils if:

- You have epilepsy
- You have a history of miscarriage
- You have heart problems

- You have diabetes
- You have blood clotting problems
- You have thyroid, liver or kidney disease

The following oils should not be used during pregnancy. This may not be a complete list, so be sure to discuss this with your doctor.

- Rosemary is thought to increase blood pressure and it may cause contractions.
- Nutmeg may have hallucinogenic effects and it can react with pain-relieving drugs in labor.
- Basil is thought to contribute to abnormal cell development.
- Jasmine and clary sage may trigger contractions.
- Sage and rose may cause bleeding in your womb.
- Juniper berry may affect your kidneys.
- Avoid laurel, thyme, angelica, cumin, citronella aniseed and cinnamon as they could stimulate contractions.
- Lavender is used to regulate periods and there is much controversy over its use during pregnancy. Do not use lavender during the first trimester.

- Clary sage can start labor so don't use this oil during pregnancy.

It's always a good idea to talk to your doctor before using essential oils.

What to Look For in Your Natural Beauty Products

Let's be honest. It can be time consuming and frustrating looking for natural beauty products that work and are safe. There are many claims on the market and yet so many products let you down. It's frustrating. All those ads and labels create so much confusion. The key is really to read the ingredients and to

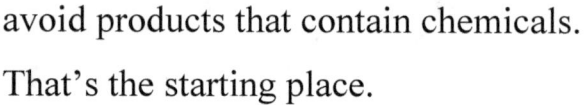 avoid products that contain chemicals. That's the starting place.

An even better option is for you to make your own products. It's really not that difficult. It's worth your time to make and use natural beauty products – your skin will love it and reward you by looking radiant and more youthful.

5 Steps to Natural Skin Care

There are five main steps to skin care.

1. Cleansing
2. Toning
3. Moisturizing
4. Exfoliating
5. Masking

That's it – five areas of care and only three of these that you have to do daily – cleanse, tone, moisturize. How simple is that. Now let's look at some recipes you can make.

Natural Recipes for Cleansing

It all begins with the cleansing that removes the dirt and grime from your face and body. Water combined with your cleanser is all you need. Here are some excellent recipes for creating your own cleanser from all natural ingredients. Use one of these natural cleanser recipes and enjoy a healthy, clean that contains no toxins.

We've given you some great recipes, but don't be afraid to get creative and make your own. Experiment a little and find the recipe that you love.

Because your cleansers contain no harsh chemical preservatives your skin will actually feel cleaner and it will definitely look healthy. You'll love the glow!

1 – Lavender & Rose Facial Cleanser

Your skin is going to feel smooth and silky. This is an excellent anti-aging cleanser.

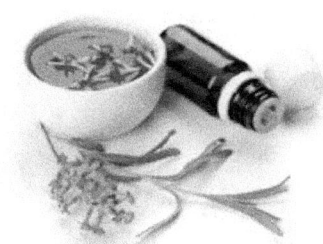

Ingredients:

- 6 drops of lavender essential oil
- 4 drops of rose essential oils
- 4 Tbsp Grapeseed oil

Instructions:

1. Pour your Grapeseed oil into a clean, dark glass bottle.
2. Add your essential oils.
3. Store in a dark, cool place.
4. Gently shake to make sure the oils are blended before you use.
5. To cleanse, apply a small amount to your face and massage into the skin.
6. Rinse with warm water.

2 - Honey & Almond Facial Cleanser for Dry Skin

Ingredients:

- 9 Tbsp whole milk
- 9 tsp honey
- 6 tsp almond oil

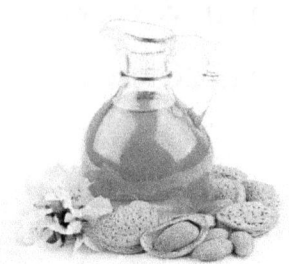

Instructions:

1. Mix ingredients in a glass bowl.
- Apply to your skin in a circular motion for 1-2 minutes.
2. Rinse with warm water.

3 - Strawberry Acne Facial Cleanser

This is excellent for all skin types.

Ingredients:

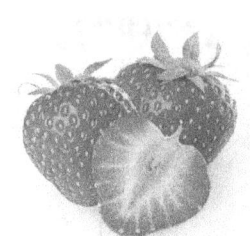

- 2 strawberries
- 6 Tbsp plain Greek yogurt

Instructions:

1. Apply to skin in a circular motion for 2 minutes.
2. Rinse with warm water.

** If you don't have fresh strawberries, you can substitute strawberry yogurt.

4 - Oily Skin Honey Exfoliating Facial Cleanser

Ingredients:

- 8 tsp honey
- 6 tsp powdered skim milk
- 3 drops of apple vinegar

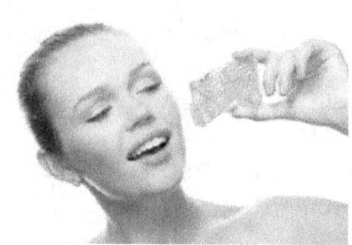

Instructions:

1. Mix the ingredients in a bowl.
2. Apply to your skin using a circular motion for 2 minutes.
3. Rinse with warm water.

5 - Cocoa Butter Facial Cleanser

Ingredients:

- 1 ½ Tbsp Grapeseed oil
- 4 Tbsp cocoa butter
- 3 drops sandalwood
- 1 tablespoons water

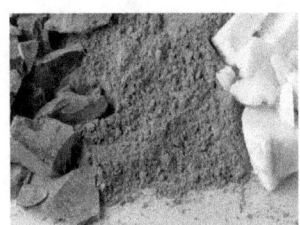

- 1 Tbsp brown sugar that you add with each wash

Instructions:

1. Melt the cocoa butter in your microwave.
2. Add water and Grapeseed oil.
3. Whisk until room temperature, then add sandalwood.
4. Store in a glass jar.
5. Add brown sugar to your hands before you wash your face.

6 - Baking Soda & Lemon Exfoliating Facial Cleanser

Ingredients:

- 2 Tbsp baking soda
- Lemon juice

Instructions:

1. In a small glass bowl, add 2 Tbsp baking soda.
2. Slowly add lemon juice until it makes make a thin, loose paste. It's going to fizz and foam.
3. Apply to your skin using a circular motion for 2 minutes.
4. Rinse with warm water.

Natural Recipes for Toning

Once you've cleansed your skin, you need to apply a toner. Applying a toner offers many benefits.

- **PH Balance** – Facial toners help balance your pH to be closer to neutral. When your pH is balanced, your skin is less likely to be oily and more likely to be smoother in appearance and glow.

- **Detox** – Facial toners will remove environmental toxins so your skin will be healthier and brighter. You'll also enjoy the long-term benefit of fewer wrinkles.

- **Shrinks Pores** – When you have larger pores, oil, dirt and toxins can become trapped, entering the skin causing infection and irritation. Facial toners will tighten your pores and your skin will look fresh and bright.

- **Acne Reduction** – Acne can cause scarring, and cause your skin to be dull, oily and unbalanced. A facial toner will remove the dead skin cells, help to reduce acne and reduce future breakouts.

- **Hydration and Nourishment** – Facial toners will hydrate your skin, which helps to maintain more youthful skin that has better elasticity and moisture.

7 - Basil Toner for Acne Skin

This recipe is a great choice if you are prone to acne. The basil acts as an antiseptic, helping to clear up acne-causing bacteria, while also improving your skin's circulation.

Ingredients:

- 6 Tbsp dried basil leaves
- 1 cup boiling water

Instructions:

1. Crush up the dried basil leaves.
2. Mix them into a cup of boiling water.
3. Once the mixture cools, strain out the leaves.
4. Put it in a glass spray bottle and spritz your skin.
5. Use a cotton ball to spread the toner gently around your face.
6. Do this daily, after cleansing.

8 – Rose Water Toner for Normal Skin

Ingredients:

- 1 Tbsp of alum
- 100 gm of rose water
- 150 gm of glycerin

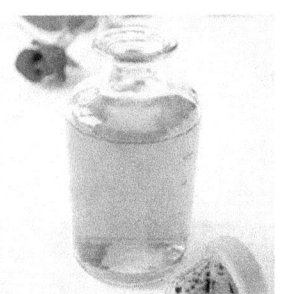

Instructions:

1. Mix all the ingredients together.
2. The rosewater toner is ready to apply.
3. Put it in a glass spray bottle and sprits your skin.
4. Use a cotton ball to spread the toner gently around your face.
5. Do this daily after cleansing.
6. Store in the refrigerator.

9 - Cucumber Toner

Ingredients:

- 2 cucumbers
- 1 cup yogurt

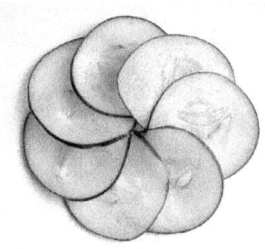

Instructions:

1. Chop up 2 medium size fresh cucumbers into fine pieces.
2. Liquidize the chopped cucumber with 1 cup of yogurt.
3. The cucumber toner is ready.
4. Apply and leave on for 10 minutes.
5. Wash off with cool water.
6. Store in the refrigerator.

10 - Dry Skin Mint Toner

Ingredients:

- 1 cup mint
- 200 gr water

Instructions:

1. Boil cup of mint in the water.
2. Put it in a glass spray bottle and spritz your skin.
3. Use a cotton ball to spread the toner gently around your face.
4. Do this daily after cleansing.
5. Store in the refrigerator.

11 - Alcohol and Alum Toner for Oily Skin

Ingredients:

- 2 tsp alcohol
- 200 gr distilled water
- 1 tsp alum

Instructions:

1. Boil water, let cool.
2. Mix alcohol with distilled water.
3. Add alum.
4. Your toning solution is ready to use.
5. Put it in a glass spray bottle and spritz your skin.
6. Use a cotton ball to spread the toner gently around your face.
7. Do this daily after cleansing.
8. Store in the refrigerator.

12 - Honey and Egg Toner

Ingredients:

- 2 eggs
- 2 tsp honey
- 2 tsp lemon juice

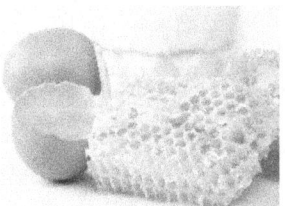

Instructions:

1. Whisk ingredients together.
2. Your toner is ready to use.
3. Put it in a glass spray bottle and spritz your skin.
4. Use a cotton ball to spread the toner gently around your face and neck. Avoid lips and eyes.
5. Leave it on for 10-15 minutes.
6. Rinse off with warm water.
7. Do this daily after cleansing.
8. Store in the refrigerator.

13 – Tea Tree and Salt Toner for Clear Skin

Ingredients:

- 4 tsp salt
- 200 ml of witch hazel
- 2 drops tea tree oil
- 5 drops lemon

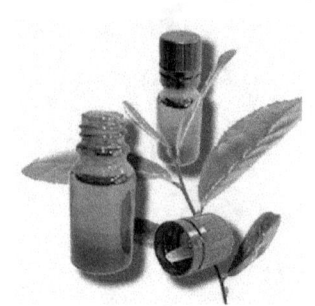

Instructions:

1. Mix salt and witch hazel.
2. Add tea tree and lemon.
3. Put it in a glass spray bottle and spritz your skin.
4. Use a cotton ball to spread the toner gently around your face.
5. Do this morning and evening after cleansing.
6. Store in the refrigerator.

Natural Recipes for Moisturizing

Moisturizing your skin is key to help you age beautifully. When your skin is moisturized, the water is trapped in the skin keeping your skin hydrated.

A moisturizer is an anti-aging must. It helps your skin retain moisture and it acts as a temporary filler for wrinkles - it makes your complexion look smooth. Your skin will look younger.

When you properly moisturize your skin, it will be more radiant and glowing. It can help to reduce dermatitis, acne and eczema. A common mistake those with oily skin or dealing with acne deal with is to think they should not moisturize. Actually, you still need to moisturize.

Not all skin moisturizers are the same. You need to make sure that you choose the right type of moisturizer for your skin type. When you are creating your own moisturizer, you have a great deal of flexibility. We've given you some great recipes. Don't be afraid to try your own recipes and create the moisturizer that's perfect for you.

14 - Avocado-Honey Moisturizer

Ingredients:

- 6 Tbsp of fresh cream
- 2 Tbsp honey
- ½ avocado

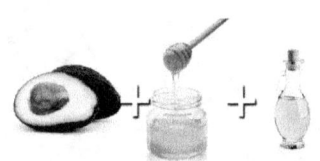

Instructions:

1. Place all three ingredients in a blender and puree into a smooth cream.
2. Apply it to your skin and leave on for at least an hour.
3. Rinse off with warm water.

15 – Beeswax & Almond Skin Cream

Ingredients:

- 2 part almond oil
- 6 parts beeswax
- 20 drops lavender essential oil

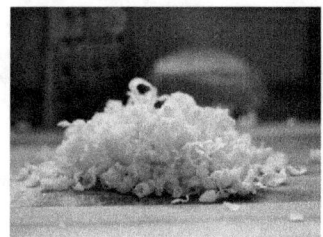

Instructions:

1. Melt the beeswax in a double boiler or microwave.
2. Mix the ingredients.
3. Pour into glass jars and let cool.
4. Use in the morning and at night.

16 - Shea Butter Cream

Ingredients:

- 1 cup coconut oil
- 1/4 cup almond oil
- 1 cup shea butter
- 20 drops of your favorite essential oil

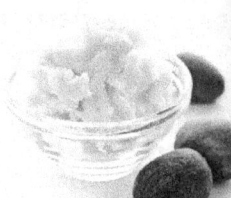

Instructions:

1. Combine the coconut oil and Shea butter on low-med heat and gently melt while mixing.
2. Once melted, add the almond oil and essential oil.
3. Mix and store in glass mason jars in the refrigerator.

17 - Dry Skin Cream

Ingredients:

- 2 1/2 Tbsp of beeswax
- ½ cup of chamomile tea
- ½ cup of almond, olive or coconut oil
- 1 ½ tsp Vitamin E

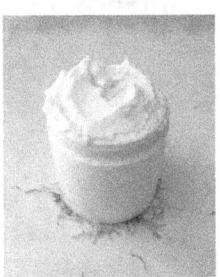

Instructions:

1. Fill a large pot with water and bring to a boil.
2. In a heat safe bowl, combine the beeswax, half the chamomile tea, and the Vitamin E.
3. Place that bowl in the pot and boil until the wax is completely melted.
4. Remove from heat.
5. Let cool for 10 minutes.
6. In your blender, pour the remaining water and slowly add the oil mixture.
7. It will start to solidify and look creamy.
8. Continue to blend.
9. Scoop into clean glass containers and cover when cool.
10. Store in refrigerator overnight. Remove from refrigerator and use daily.

18 - Nourishing Facial Serum

Ingredients:

1. 2 Tbsp Jojoba oil
2. 1 tsp Evening Primrose oil
3. 3 drops Geranium essential oil
4. 2 drops Carrot Seed essential oil
5. 3 drops Neroli essential oil
6. 3 drops Frankincense essential oil

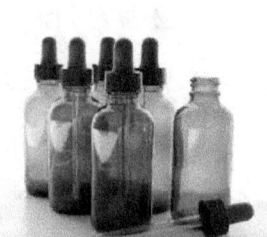

Instructions:

1. Combine the ingredients in a dark glass bottle with a dropper.
2. Shake for 2-3 minutes.
3. Use only 1-2 drops of serum over the entire face and neck area.

19 - Anti Aging Wrinkle Face Serum

Ingredients:

- 8 Tbsp extra virgin olive oil
- 20 drops of one of the following essential oils: frankincense, myrrh, rose, patchouli or lavender.

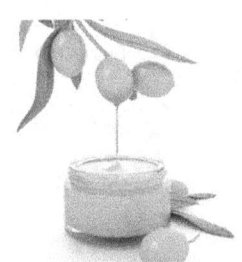

Instructions:

1. Massage a small amount of the oil into your face and neck at bedtime.

20 - Anti Aging Mango Butter Cream

Ingredients:

- 8 Tbsp beeswax
- 6 Tbsp mango butter
- 15 Tbsp coconut oil
- 20 drops carrot seed essential oil

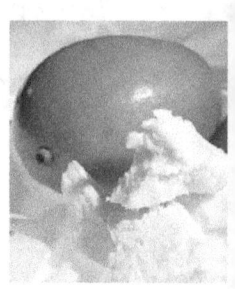

Instructions:

1. Melt wax and butter together.
2. Add the oil.
3. Stir well and let cool.
4. Before the lotion sets add the essential oil.
5. Mix until completely smooth.
6. Pour into a glass jar, let harden and seal.

21 - Mature Skin Lotion

Ingredients:

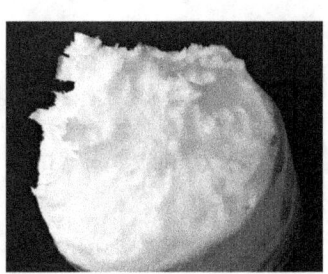

- 5 oz beeswax
- 12 oz jojoba oil
- 16 drops carrot seed essential oil
- 16 drops myrrh
- 20 drops frankincense
- 20 drops lavender

Instructions:

1. Melt ingredients together.
2. Once melted blend thoroughly
3. Let cool to about lukewarm, then add essential oils.
4. Cool completely.

Natural Recipes for Exfoliating

Exfoliating is a very important part in caring for your skin. It sloughs away dead skin cells and it unclogs the dirt and oils that become trapped in your pores. Exfoliate no more than three times a week.

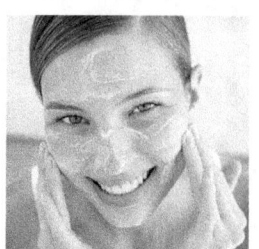

Exfoliating has a number of benefits:

- It will keep skin soft and glowing
- It will remove the dead skin and stop your pores from clogging, which can help to control acne.
- Speeds up the skins natural renewal process.
- It helps the moisturizer penetrate the skin deeper.
- Even skin tone by removing dead skin cells that cause discoloration.
- Leads to skin that is visibly brighter.
- It reduces fine lines and wrinkles.

These exfoliating recipes will keep your skin healthy and glowing.

22 - Sugar n Spice Face Scrub

Ingredients:

- 4 Tbsp granulated sugar
- 4 Tbsp dark brown sugar
- 4 Tbsp almond oil
- 3 tsp pure vanilla extract
- 4 Tbsp ground oatmeal
- 1 tsp cinnamon

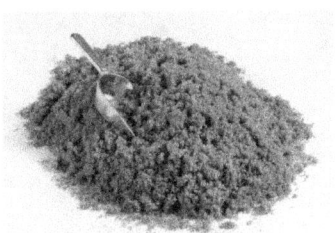

Instructions:

1. Combine and mix all ingredients.
2. Scrub your face with the mixture for 1-2 minutes.
3. Rinse with warm water.

23 - Baking Soda Scrub

1. Make a paste of just baking soda and water.
2. Gently rub it onto your skin and leave it on for 5 to 10 minutes
3. Rinse off.

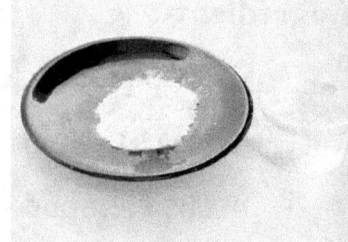

24 - Sugar Scrub

1. Combine 2 tsp sugar with 1 tsp honey and a squeeze of fresh lemon juice.
2. Mix well.
3. Add more sugar if you find it too lose.

4. Gently rub it onto your skin and leave it on for 5 to 10 minutes.
5. Rinse off.

25 - Coffee Scrub

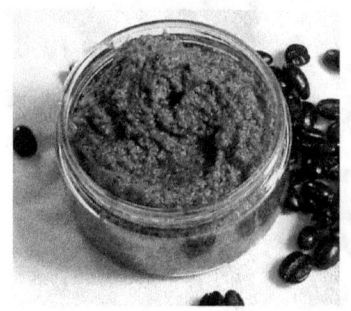

1. Combine 2 Tbsp of ground coffee with 2 Tbsp olive oil.
2. Gently rub it onto your skin and leave it on for 5 to 10 minutes.
3. Rinse off.

26 - Oatmeal Scrub

Oatmeal exfoliates and it absorbs and removes dirt and impurities.

1. Combine 1 tablespoon of ground oatmeal with 1/4 teaspoon of salt and 1 teaspoon of olive oil to make it into a paste.

2. Gently rub it onto your skin in circular motions.
3. Let sit for 10 minutes.
4. Rinse with warm water.

27 - Lemon Sugar Face Scrub

Ingredients:

- ¼ cup lemon juice
- 1 ½ Tbsp table salt
- Sugar

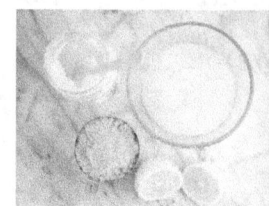

Instructions:

1. Mix the ingredients and add sugar until the mixture is thick.
2. Apply to damp face.
3. Let sit 5 minutes.
4. Scrub using gentle circular motions.
5. Rinse well with warm water. Your skin will be smooth and so soft.

28 – Honey & Sugar Facial Scrub

Ingredients:

- 6 Tbsp Milk
- Approx. 3 cups white sugar
- 4 tsp olive oil
- 4 Tbsp honey

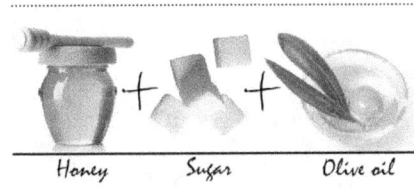

Honey   Sugar   Olive oil

Instructions:

1. Mix all the ingredients until it is a smooth consistency and not runny. Add more sugar if necessary.
2. Apply to dry face in a circular motion.
3. Wash off with warm water then follow with cold water.
4. Pat dry
5. Store extra in the refrigerator in a glass container.

29 – The Simple Baking Soda Body Exfoliator

This is a quick and easy way to exfoliate your
entire body. Keep a container of baking soda
in the shower.

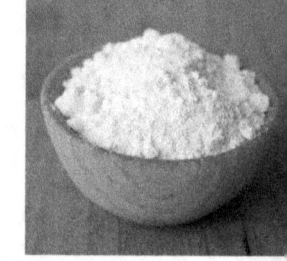

Take a tablespoon of baking soda and apply
starting with your face working down your body in circular
motions. Rinse with warm water.

30 – The Cane Sugar Body Exfoliator

Sugar is a natural source of glycolic acid boosting new cell production, breaking down the protein the holds the dead cells onto your skin.

Mix cane sugar with your olive oil to form a paste. Scrub beginning with your face in a circular motion, working down your body. Rinse with warm water.

31 – The Sea Salt Body Exfoliator

Sea salt is full of trace minerals rejuvenating the skin and stimulating cell growth. It's an excellent choice for dry skin. Mix the sea salt with your almond oil and a couple of drops of lavender oil to form a paste. In a circular motion, scrub beginning with your face and working down your body. Rinse with warm water.

32 – The Oatmeal Body Exfoliator

Oatmeal is a gentle exfoliator that's excellent for sensitive skin.
Mix fine oatmeal with honey and a
tablespoon of yogurt to form a
paste.

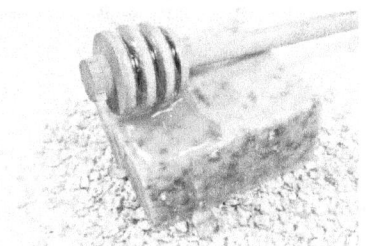

In a circular motion, scrub
beginning with your face and working down your body. Leave
on for 30 minutes. Rinse with warm water.

33 – The Kefir Body Exfoliator

Kefir is like yogurt. In fact, if you don't have kefir you can substitute yogurt.

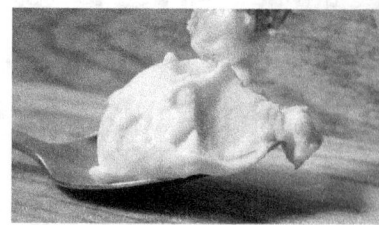

In a circular motion, scrub beginning with your face and working down your body. Leave on for 30 minutes. Rinse with warm water. Your skin will be soft and smooth.

34 – Sweet Almond Facial Scrub

Ingredients:

- 6 Tbsp of fresh cream
- 1 ½ cups of brown sugar
- 2 cups of white sugar
- ¾ cup of ground almonds
- 4 Tbsp olive oil

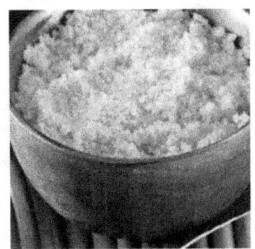

Instructions:

1. Mix all ingredients.
2. In a circular motion, apply the mixture to your dry face.
3. Wash your face using warm water, followed by cold water.
4. Pat dry.
5. Store in a glass jar and store in the refrigerator.

35 – The Better Than Botox Facial Scrub

Ingredients:

- 2 Tbsp baking soda
- 2 Tbsp raw Manuka honey
- 2 drops lavender essential oil
- 2 drops geranium essential oil
- 2 drops frankincense essential oil

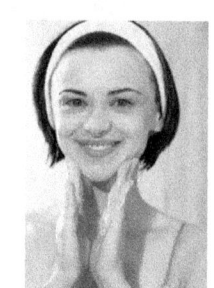

Instructions:

1. Combine the baking soda and honey together until it looks like a paste.
2. Add the essential oils.
3. Place a warm washcloth on your face for a minute to open up your pores.
4. Gently rub your face using small circular motions for 3-5 minutes to fully remove the dead skin from your face and allow the essential oils to work their magic.
5. Rinse off with warm water.
6. Use this scrub no more than twice a week.

This scrub is alkaline to the skin, so to even out your pH splash your face with rosewater afterwards. This will naturally balance your skin

Natural Recipes for Face Masks

A face mask will remove surface dirt and grime, as well as, draw out impurities. Face masks are important in your anti aging treatments. A few of the benefits of using a face mask include.

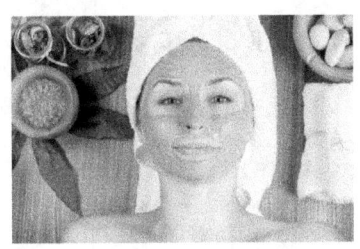

- It can help you to develop more refined pores and clearer skin.
- It deep cleanses the pores and removes dead skin cells.
- It removes oily substances that can clog your pores.
- It improves hydration. The water from the mask penetrates deep into the skin's epidermis.
- It softens the skin and improves elasticity.
- It reduces fine lines and wrinkles.
- It helps to even out the skin tone.
- It firms the skin.

Let's look at some easy to make at home face masks

36 - Regenerative Face Mask

Ingredients:

- 8 Tbsp of natural green clay
- 10 drops of one of the following essential oils: lavender, frankincense, tea tree oil, or rosemary.
- Water

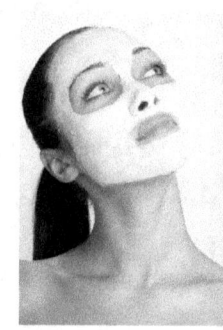

Instructions:

1. Add enough water to make a paste.
2. Apply evenly to your face and neck.
3. Leave 30-40 minutes
4. Rinse with cool water.
5. Pat dry and moisturize.
6. Repeat once a week.

37 – Cucumber & Yogurt Facial Mask

Ingredients:

- 1 peeled cucumber
- 8 tsp plain yogurt
- 4 Tbsp instant nonfat dry milk

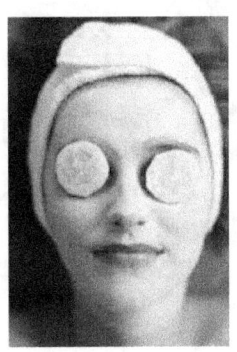

Instructions:

1. Put everything in the blender and mix until smooth.
2. Apply to your face but avoid the eye area.
3. Leave on for 30 minutes.
4. Rinse off with warm water.

38 – Anti Wrinkle Face Mask

Ingredients:

- 4 Tbsp olive oil
- 3 Tbsp milk
- 1 Tbsp carrot juice
- 5 Tbsp Yogurt

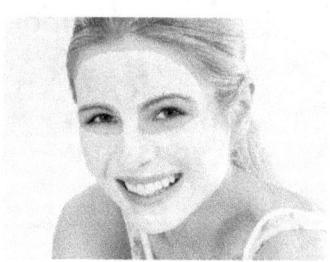

Instructions:

1. Combine the ingredients.
2. Apply to face and allow to set for 10-15 minutes.
3. Wash off with warm water.
4. Great for moisturizing tired, dry skin.

39 – Sweet as Honey Face Mask

Ingredients:

- 2 eggs
- 5 Tbsp powdered milk
- 4 Tbsp honey

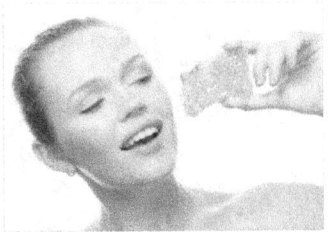

Instructions:

1. Mix all ingredients well until they are smooth and creamy

2. Apply evenly on your face.

3. Let sit for 15 to 20 minutes.

4. Rinse with lukewarm water followed by cold water.

40 - Avocado Honey Moisturizing Mask

Ingredients:

- 1 very ripe avocado
- 1 ½ cups honey

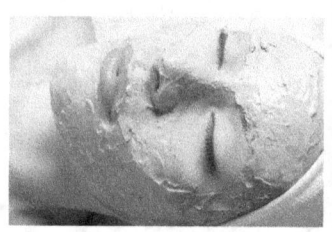

Instructions:

1. Mash avocado in honey with fork until smooth.
2. Apply to your clean, dry face.
3. Let sit for 15 minutes.
4. Rinse well with warm water.
5. Pat dry.

41 - Apple Honey Face Mask

Ingredients:

- 1 medium size apple
- 8 Tbsp honey

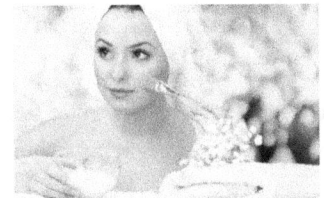

Instructions:

1. Grate apple very fine.
2. Mix together the grated apple and honey.
3. Smooth over the skin.
4. Leave on for 15 minutes.
5. Rinse off with cool water.

42 - Cucumber & Yogurt Face Mask

Ingredients:

- 4 Tbsp finely ground oatmeal
- 4 Tbsp brewer's yeast
- 1 ½ whole cucumber
- 5 Tbsp plain yogurt or sour cream
- 3 tsp honey

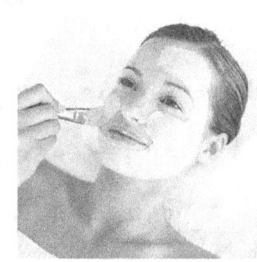

Instructions:

1. Mix yeast and oats and set aside.
2. Process the peeled cucumber.
3. Mix in the yogurt and honey.
4. Add the brewer's yeast and oats.
5. Process until smooth.
6. Apply to your face.
7. Leave on for 20 minutes.
8. Rinse off.

43 - Clay Face Mask Recipe for Normal Skin

Ingredients:

- 4 teaspoon water
- 4 Tbsp green clay
- 2 egg yolks
- 4 drops geranium essential oil

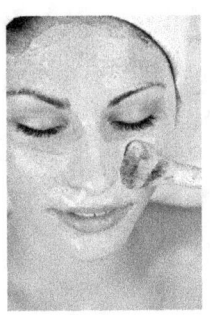

Instructions:

1. Mix all ingredients.
2. Apply to face.
3. Leave on 20 minutes.
4. Wash your face with warm water.

Natural Recipes for Fighting Age Spots

Age spots are something most of us face as we age. In fact, your hands are a dead giveaway of your age. These natural recipes will help to fade your age spots.

44 - Lemon-Agave Age Spot Fighter

Ingredients:

- 1 cup cooked rice
- 2 Tbsp agave nectar
- 2 Tbsp lemon juice

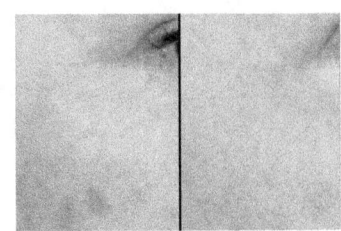

Instructions:

1. Mix all ingredients together and blend.
2. Apply the mixture onto your dry hands in a circular motion for 1-2 minutes.
3. Rinse with warm water.

45 – Horseradish Age Spot Remover

Ingredients:

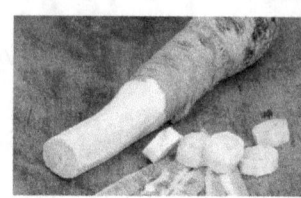

- ½ tsp lemon juice
- 2 tsp horseradish
- 1 tsp vinegar
- 6 drops rosemary essential oil

Instructions:

1. Mix all ingredients together and blend.
2. Apply to age spots using cotton ball.
3. Leave on for 10 minutes.
4. Rinse with warm water.

46 - Aloe Vera Age Spot Remover for Mature Skin

Ingredients:

- 4 ounces Aloe vera gel
- 4 ounces orange blossom water
- 21 tsp vinegar
- 12 drops rose geranium essential oil
- 8 drops frankincense essential oil
- 4 drops carrot seed essential oil
- 1600 IU vitamin E oil

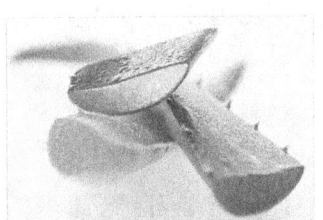

Instructions:

1. Mix ingredients.
2. Apply as needed.
3. Rinse with warm water.

Body Butters

Body butters play an important part in your skin care regimes too. After all, you want your entire body to be soft and supple, and you want your skin to age gracefully.

When you use your body butters regularly, you'll really enjoy the benefits. This is especially true when you make these butters yourself. They have no harmful chemicals and are packed with the most powerful nutrients around.

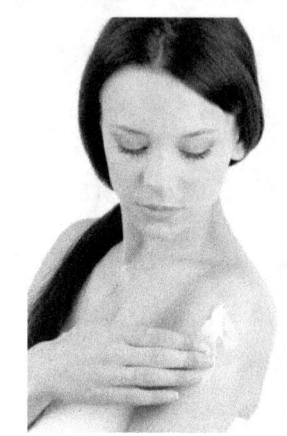

Here are some fabulous natural recipes for body butters that you are going to love.

47 - Vanilla Body Butter

This body butter that smells so good and it deeply moisturizes your skin, while soothing your soul.

Ingredients:

- 3 cup raw cocoa butter
- 1 ½ cups sweet almond oil
- 1 ½ cups coconut oil
- 6 vanilla beans

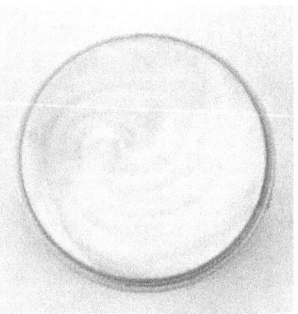

Instructions:

1. On medium heat in a double boiler, melt the cocoa butter and coconut oil.
2. Once it is melted, remove from the heat and let cool for 30 minutes.
3. Grind your vanilla beans.
4. Stir the sweet almond oil and vanilla bean bits into the cocoa butter and coconut oil.
5. Place it in the freezer for about 30 minutes to chill. Wait until oils start to partially solidify.

6. Whip with an electric mixer until it is butter-like consistency.
7. Spoon it into your glass jar(s). It makes about 5 cups of whipped butter. Store it in the refrigerator.

You'll feel sexy and sensual. You can apply it before bedtime to improve your sleep.

48 - Key Lime Body Butter

This body butter smells so good you might want to eat it. It works great on dry spots like your elbows and heels.

Ingredients:

- 1 Tbsp macadamia nut oil (or olive oil if you don't have macadamia nut)
- 2 cups coconut oil
- 2 Tbsp Aloe Vera gel
- 20 drops lime essential oil
- 20 drops lemon essential oil

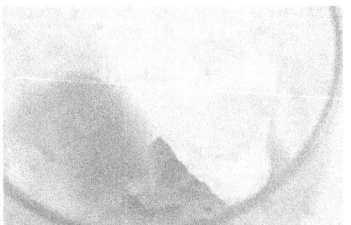

Instructions:

1. Place all of your ingredients into a glass mixing bowl. Don't melt the coconut oil first because it has to be solid to whip up.
2. Use your electric mixer and whip it into a light, airy uniformity.
3. Spoon your body butter into a glass jar and seal.
4. Store at room temperature.

49 - Peppermint & Chocolate Body Butter

This is a great body butter for the hot season, because it has a high melting point. The peppermint oil in the whipped butter makes this refreshing and cool in the summer heat.

Ingredients:

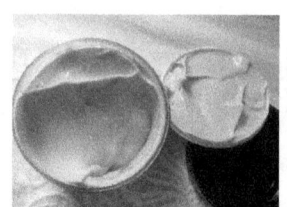

- 2 cups cocoa butter
- 2 cups coconut oil
- 80 drops peppermint essential oil

Instructions:

1. Add the cocoa butter and coconut into a double boiler.
2. On medium heat, while stirring constantly until they both have completely melted.
3. Cool the mixture in your refrigerator until it is mostly solid.
4. Sprinkle about 80 drops of peppermint essential oil on top.
5. Mix for 5-10 minutes until the body butter is whipped and airy.
6. Scoop into a glass jar and seal.
7. Store in the refrigerator.

50 – Mint & Shea Body Butter

Peppermint is soothing. Add the shea butter and you'll love it!

Ingredients:

  1 cup of shea butter

  ½ cup tallow

  ½ cup of jojoba oil

  ½ tsp peppermint essential oil

  1 Tbsp Vitamin E oil

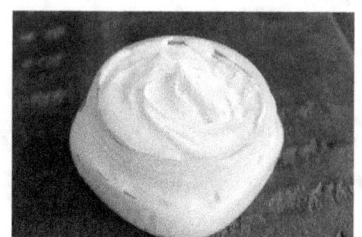

Instructions:

1. Use a double boiler to gently heat the shea butter and tallow until they are completely melted.
2. Remove the bowl from heat and stir in the jojoba oil.
3. Set up an ice bath and let it chill for 5 minutes.
4. Stir in the peppermint essential oil and Vitamin E oil.
5. Keep it chilling in the ice bath until it is thoroughly chilled.
6. Whip using a mixer until it forms stiff peaks.
7. Scoop the mixture into glass jars and then seal. It should last for about 12 months.

51 – Cocoa & Cinnamon Whipped Body Butter

This body butter smells so good – it's the cacao powder, nutmeg and cinnamon – yummy!

Ingredients:

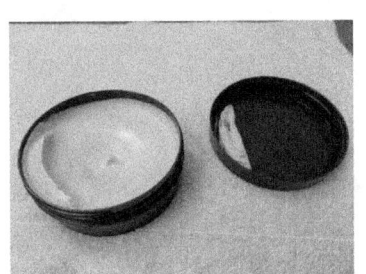

1 cup coconut oil

1 cup shea butter

1 cup almond oil or jojoba oil

3 Tbsp cocoa

1 Tbsp ground nutmeg

4 Tbsp ground cinnamon

1600 IU Vitamin E oil

20 drops of your favorite essential oil

Instructions:

1. Using a double boiler and on low-medium heat, melt your coconut oil.
2. Once they are completely melted you can remove from the heat.
3. Let stand to cool for 30 minutes.
4. Mix in the almond oil, cocoa powder, essential oil, cinnamon, nutmeg and Vitamin E.
5. Place the oil mixture in the freezer and let it firm up.

6. Once the oil mixture is partially solidified, remove it from the freezer.

7. Whip until it forms peaks that resemble whipped butter.

8. Scoop into glass jars and seal. It should last 6 - 12 months.

Lip Exfoliator and Lip Balm

Taking care of your lips is as important as taking care of your skin. After all, your lips are exposed to the same conditions as the rest of your skin. These natural recipes will keep your lips soft and supple.

52 - Java Lip Exfoliator

This easy to make recipe will slough dry, dead skin from your lips makes them look instantly plumper and pinker.

Ingredients:

- ½ teaspoon of coconut oil
- ¼ teaspoon fresh coffee grounds
- ¼ teaspoon Kosher salt

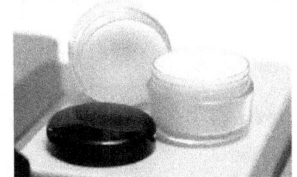

Instructions:

1. Mix ingredients well in a bowl.
2. Apply to entire your mouth and massage for about 5 minutes.
3. Wipe clean with a warm wet washcloth.

53 - Lip Balm

This is such an easy lip balm to make and it's great for

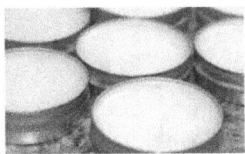 chapped lips or dry hands. Because it's made from coconut oil and beeswax, it is very tasty.

Ingredients:

- 2 parts coconut oil
- 1 part beeswax
- 2 drops Vitamin E

Instructions:

1. Mix ingredients well in a bowl.
2. Press into container and store in refrigerator.

54 – Coconut & Rose Lip Balm

Ingredients:

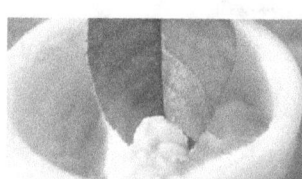

- ¼ cup Coconut Oil
- ¼ cup Beeswax
- ¼ cup Shea Butter
- 2 tsp Vanilla Extract
- ½ cup Rose Petals (fresh or dried)
- 2 tsp Sweet Almond Oil

Instructions:

1. Mix all ingredients into a small saucepan.
2. Heat on low until everything is melted, or use the microwave.
3. Pour into containers for storage.
4. Let cool completely.

55 - Minty Lip Balm

This is perfect for those cold, dry winter days.

Ingredients:

- 6 drops peppermint oil
- 4 Tbsp almond oil
- 2 Tbsp beeswax pellets

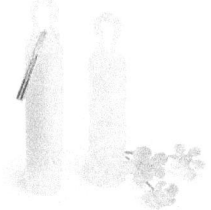

Instructions:

1. Put the two tablespoons almond oil and one tablespoon beeswax in a glass jar and close the lid.
2. Heat the jar in a pot with water on medium-high heat until the wax is completely melted.
3. Remove the jar and stir your mixture, adding your peppermint oil. More peppermint is not necessarily better as it can cause your lips to burn. So if you want a more minty taste experiment with one drop at a time.
4. Pour the mixture into your containers. Let stand for two hours until hard.

56 – Hemp & Honey Lip Balm

The Manuka honey makes this an excellent lip balm. In addition to softening your lips, it has antibacterial properties.

Ingredients:

- 15 drops citrus essential oil
- 30 gr beeswax
- 2 gr carnauba wax
- 15 gr cocoa butter
- 10 gr shea butter
- 1 oz almond oil
- ½ oz hemp oil
- 1 oz manuka honey

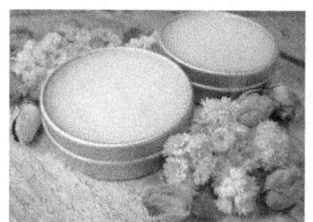

Instructions:

1. Melt the beeswax, cocoa butter, almond oil, shea butter and carnauba wax in the double boiler.
2. Add in your honey and hemp oil, stirring constantly until it is liquid. Honey is not soluble with oil, so to completely dissolve it you will need to mix with a milk frothier.

3. Remove from heat, add essential oils and blend with the frothier while the mixture cools.

4. Pour into tubes and leave to set.

Hair Shampoo and Conditioner

What would a book of natural recipes be without some hair shampoo and conditioner options? You want your hair to be as healthy as your skin. The benefits of using natural shampoos and conditioners that you create include:

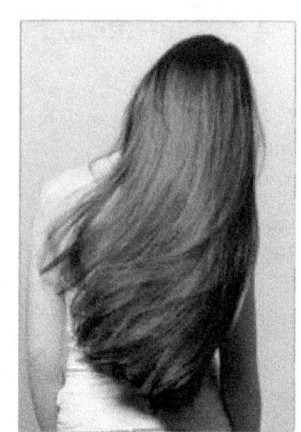

- **No Isopropyl Alcohol** – This petroleum-derived substance dissolves oils. It is found in commercial products like shellac and antifreeze. It is very drying and removes moisture from your hair, which damages your hair.

- **Propylene Glycol** – It helps ingredients in your shampoo to penetrate your hair. The trouble is it breaks down healthy-hair proteins and it can irritate the eyes and skin, especially if you have sensitive skin.

- **No Sulfates** - Sulfates are strong chemical detergents. They are commonly used in kitchen and automotive degreasers. They make your shampoo foam, but they are known to irritate the scalp, causing itching and redness.

- **Formaldehyde** – This chemical preservative is a known carcinogen that kills bacteria and irritates the respiratory system. It can also cause skin inflammation.

Why not create your own natural shampoos and conditioners with these recipes.

57 – The Easy as 123 Shampoo

This might be a really simple recipe, but it is still highly effective.

Ingredients:

- 2 Tbsp baking soda
- 2 cups water

Instructions:

Mix and pour into bottles. It's that simple. When you wash your hair give the bottle a good shake and then squirt it directly onto your scalp. Massage gently for a couple of minutes and rinse.

58 - Coconut Deep Conditioner

This recipe will keep your hair hydrated, smooth and shiny. Use weekly.

Ingredients:

- ½ cup mayonnaise
- 3 Tbsp coconut oil
- 3 drops favorite essential oil

If you have long hair, you may need more. Just double the recipe or triple it if you need.

Instructions:

1. Mix ingredients together.
2. Apply and cover your scalp with a plastic wrap.
3. Leave on for at least 30 minutes.
4. Rinse hair thoroughly.

59 - Avocado Conditioner

This monthly treatment is rich in Vitamins A and B. It will keep in your refrigerator for a week.

Ingredients:

- 2 very ripe avocados
- 1 cup mayonnaise or you can use coconut milk

Instructions:

1. Mash the avocados
2. Mix with mayonnaise or coconut milk to form a paste.
3. Comb through hair and cover your head with a towel.
4. Leave on for 30 minutes.
5. Rinse, shampoo, and rinse.

60 - Super Shine Rinse

Instructions:

Use to remove build-up. You can use it weekly on most hair types. The shelf life is 6 months.

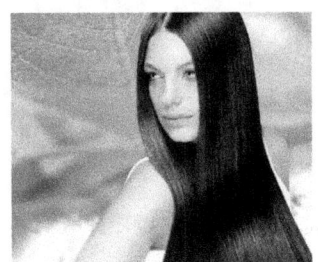

Instructions:

- ½ cup apple cider vinegar
- 30 cups water

Instructions:

Combine ingredients the ingredients, mix and pour into bottle. Use every couple of weeks. Wash hair, rinse, leave in for 30 minutes, and rinse your hair with cool water.

61 - Avocado Hair Paste

This is great for your hair. It will keep it healthy and shiny. You can use it monthly. It will last a week if refrigerated.

Ingredients:

2 over ripe avocados

3 tsp lemon juice

2 tsp sea salt

1 tsp pure aloe juice or gel

Instructions:

1. Mash the avocados and combine ingredients into a paste.
2. Comb through your hair and cover your head with a towel.
3. Leave on for at least 30 minutes.
4. Rinse, shampoo, and rinse again.

62 - Herbal Tea Shampoo

This works great with an apple cider vinegar rinse. It lasts for a month in the refrigerator.

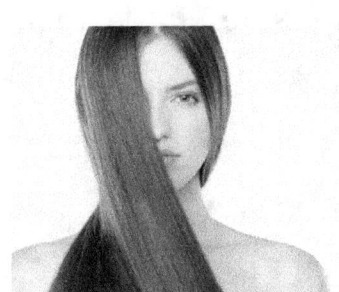

Ingredients:

- 1 cup distilled water
- 2 Tbsp peppermint
- 2 Tbsp lavender
- 2 Tbsp Nettle
- 2 Tbsp Rosemary
- ½ cup vegetable glycerin or castile soap
- 1 tsp salt
- 1 tsp witch hazel
- 10 drops of lavender or ylang ylang

Instructions:

1. Boil water and use a combination of the dried herbs to make a tea.
2. Steep the tea and let it cool, then add the rest of the ingredients.
3. Mix and pour into a bottle.

63 - Lavender and Rosemary Hair Oil

For best results, leave in overnight. It lasts for 2 weeks.

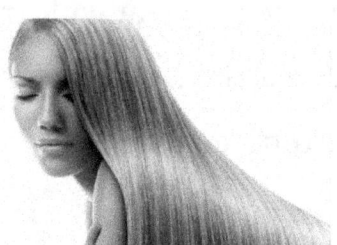

Ingredients:

- 4 drops lavender essential oil
- 3 drops rosemary essential oil
- 1 tsp olive oil

Instructions:

1. Mix together and let mellow a few hours to blend.
2. Warm in the microwave and massage into your scalp and hair, then wrap with a towel and leave on for an hour.
3. Wash and rinse with warm, then rinse with cold.

You can also put a couple of drops on your hands and run it through your hair any time.

64 – Mayo & Egg Conditioner

Ingredients:

- 1 cup plain yogurt
- 1 cup mayonnaise
- 2 egg whites

Instructions:

1. Mix ingredients together.
2. Lather into your hair with a focus on your ends. Make sure all strands are well coated.
3. Put a shower cap on or wrap in plastic and leave on for 1 hour.
4. Rinse really well because of the egg, it can take a little effort but it's worth it.

You Are Ready to Make it Your Own

That's it – now really it wasn't all that bad, was it? It's actually pretty exciting to know that with just a few ingredients, most of 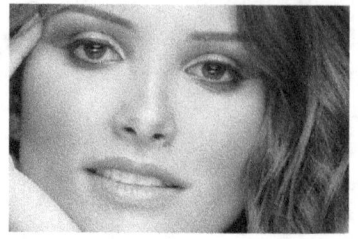 which, you likely have in your kitchen; you can make superior skin care products that will leave your skin soft and supple. You can be proud, knowing that your skin will age gently and gracefully without chemicals that have the potential to cause serious health risks, like cancer.

When it comes to your skin care, you are now in the driver's seat and ready to make it on your own. Feels pretty good doesn't it?

Now the next challenge is to turn to natural cosmetics. Whether you decide to make them or buy them, this next step will offer you additional protection from the chemicals that have made themselves part of our everyday life. Contrary to what the beauty industry would like us to believe, putting chemicals on our skin daily can be dangerous.

You're beautiful inside and out. Remember that healthy skin isn't achieved just by what you put on the outside. It's also important to eat a healthy diet and exercise regularly. Lifestyle choices are important. These combined with the use of natural skin care products will help you to be the best you can be and look your very best.

Bonus Recipes

You have 64 natural beauty recipes already and now you'll have more with these bonus recipes. Have fun and enjoy!

65 - All Natural Homemade Eye Shadow

Ingredients:

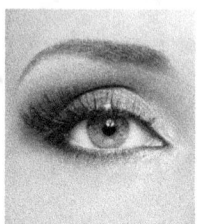

For the base:

- Shea butter
- Arrowroot powder

Combine any of these:

- Nutmeg
- Cocoa powder
- Dried beet powder
- Allspice
- Turmeric

Color Options:

<u>Golden Brown:</u>

- ½ tsp arrowroot powder
- ¾ tsp nutmeg

- ¼ tsp turmeric
- ½ tsp shea butter

Pale Pink:

- ½ tsp arrowroot powder
- ½ tsp dried beet powder
- ¼ tsp cocoa powder
- ½ tsp shea butter

Mauve:

- ½ tsp arrowroot powder
- ¾ tsp allspice
- ¾ tsp dried beet powder
- ¼ tsp cocoa powder
- ½ tsp shea butter

Light Brown:

- ½ tsp arrowroot
- ½ tsp cocoa powder
- ½ tsp shea butter

Instructions:

1. Place ½-1 tsp of arrowroot powder in a small bowl. The more arrowroot powder you use the lighter the color of the eye shadow.
2. Add your other powders or spices and mix thoroughly until you get the color you want.
3. Once you have your color, you can add in approx. ½ tsp of shea butter.
4. Cream the butter in with the powder until you have a soft, creamy powder. Shea butter helps your homemade eye shadow stay on and it's nice and moisturizing.

66 - Homemade Foundation Powder

Ingredients:

- Arrowroot powder
- Ground cinnamon
- Cocoa powder
- Nutmeg
- Almond oil

Instructions:

1. Start with your arrowroot powder as your base. You will need 1 tablespoon for light skin and 1 teaspoon for dark skin.

2. Slowly add in one or a combination of the cinnamon, nutmeg, and/or cocoa powder until you get the shade and tone of foundation you want.

3. If you prefer a foundation that's more compact, you can add more almond oil to the mixture and press down into a compact. Begin with 3 drops and continue to add until you get the texture you want.

4. Use a brush to apply this homemade foundation.

67 - Natural Homemade Mascara

Ingredients:

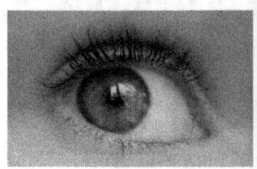

- 8 tsp aloe vera gel
- 4 tsp coconut oil
- 2 capsules of activated charcoal (for black) or cocoa powder (for brown)
- A clean mascara container
- 1 tsp grated bees wax

Instructions:

1. Put the aloe vera gel, grated beeswax and coconut oil in a small saucepan on low heat.
2. Stir until everything is melted.
3. Open 2 capsules of activated charcoal or cocoa powder depending on color you want and pour into your oil mixture.
4. Stir until fully blended.
5. Remove from heat.
6. Pour into a small plastic bag, and then roll the bag, forcing the mixture down to the bottom. Cut a tiny hole in the opposite corner of the bag.

7. Keep the small-hole-end securely in your mascara tube. Start to work the mixture into the tube. Go slow. When you are done, twist the wand on tightly.

Like any mascara, dispose of the tube and brush after 4 - 6 months. If it starts to smell different or pungent, get rid of it.

68 – Natural Homemade Blush

Ingredients:

- Hibiscus powder
- Arrowroot powder
- Cinnamon (optional)

Instructions:

1. Start with about 1 Tbsp arrowroot powder.
2. Add the hibiscus powder a little at a time until you get the color you want.
3. For a little depth, add a little cinnamon.

69 - Homemade Eye Liner

Ingredients:

- 8 tsp aloe vera gel
- 4 tsp coconut oil
- 3 capsules of activated charcoal for black or 1 tsp cocoa powder for brown

Instructions:

1. Thoroughly mix all ingredients.
2. Store in an airtight container in a dark/cool place.
3. Use a clean brush to ensure you don't introduce any bacteria to the mixture.

70 - Dye Your Hair Using Coffee!

Ingredients:

1. 1 cup conditioner
2. 8 Tbsp instant coffee

Instructions:

1. Mix the coffee and conditioner together. Keep mixing until the coffee has dissolved.

2. Put a towel around your shoulders; dip your fingers in the mixture (you might want to wear disposable gloves). Work it through your hair evenly. It's best to start with your roots.

3. Once you have applied all of the dye, if you have longer hair clip your hair up so you don't drip on anything.

4. You need to leave it on for at 75 minutes.

5. Rinse your hair. Do not shampoo. When the water runs clear, you can stop.

6. Style in your usual way.

- If you have long hair use more conditioner and more coffee.

- If you have lots of gray, you can repeat the process a couple of days in a row.

- If you drip dye on you or your things, it doesn't stain.

- This is not for blonde-haired people.

- To keep the results you'll need to do this once a week.

71 - Natural Deodorant Recipe

Ingredients:

- 1/3 cup coconut oil
- 1/4 cup baking soda
- 1/4 cup arrowroot powder
- 4 tablespoons cornstarch
- Essential oils–try tea tree, lavender, sweet orange, or frankincense

Instructions:

1. Mix baking soda, cornstarch and arrowroot powder in a bowl.
2. Add coconut oil and use a fork to blend into the dry ingredients.
3. Add 5-10 drops of your chosen essential oil.
4. Add more coconut oil or baking soda to achieve your desired consistency.

72 - Coconut Oil Tooth Scrub

Ingredients:

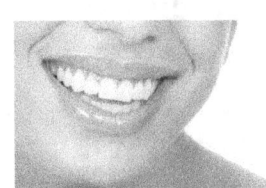

- 4 tbsp coconut oil
- 2 tbsp bentonite clay
- 2 tbsp baking soda
- 1/2 tsp natural green stevia
- 10 drops of peppermint essential oil

Instructions:

1. Combine all ingredients until smooth and blended
2. You may add more coconut oil or dry ingredients to create a paste with a texture you prefer.
3. To use, just spread a small amount of tooth scrub on your toothbrush and brush your teeth like you would with toothpaste.
4. Store in an airtight container.

73 - Homemade Mouthwash that Whitens and Remineralizes

Ingredients:

- 3 cups of filtered water
- 1 ½ teaspoon xylitol crystals
- 2 teaspoons calcium carbonate powder
- 15 drops concentrated trace minerals liquid
- 8 drops spearmint essential oil
- 15 drops peppermint essential oil
- 5 drops lemon essential oil

Instructions:

1. In a glass mixing cup, stir together the xylitol crystals and the calcium powder.
2. Add the essential oils and the liquid minerals.
3. Add water and mix well.
4. Pour into a glass bottle and seal tightly.
5. Shake ingredients together for about a minute to make sure that the xylitol dissolves.
6. Always give is a good shake before you use it.
7. Store in the refrigerator for up to two weeks.

74 - Hair Mousse for Healthy Curls

Ingredients:

- ½ cup Shea butter, warmed slightly to soften
- ¼ cup coconut oil
- ¼ cup olive oil
- 20 drops lavender essential oil
- 15 drops tea tree essential oil
- 35 drops eucalyptus essential oil

Instructions:

1. Place the shea butter and coconut oil in a bowl and mix.
2. Beat on medium-high until light and fluffy - takes about 10 minutes.
3. Add the essential oils, turn the mixer back on medium-high, and slowly pour the olive oil in until all has been mixed in.
4. Keep mixing for about 3 minutes.
5. Store in a cool, dark place.

75 – Homemade Bar Soap

Ingredients:

- 20 oz frozen canned coconut milk
- 6 oz lye
- 20 oz lard
- 20 oz coconut oil
- 1 oz of essential oil

Instructions:

1. In a glass bowl, mix the coconut milk and lye. Use a wooden spoon.
2. In a saucepan over medium heat, melt the lard, coconut oil and essential oil to 115 degrees.
3. Slowly add the oil mixture and lye mixture together. Using a hand blender blend until thickened. (at least 10 minutes)
4. Pour the mixture into your molds and dry for 18 to 24 hours.
5. Remove from the molds, slice into bars, and place on racks to dry for 4 weeks to allow for saponification.

DIY homemade beauty product recipes... Dare to explore and create beautiful, healthy skin using products that are natural and chemical free. Happy hunting!

www.ingramcontent.com/pod-product-compliance
Lightning Source LLC
Chambersburg PA
CBHW062008280526
45787CB00005B/2022